MW01172854

S.L. NEWMAN

Energy Boost

How Small Changes And The Right Habits Can Boost Your Energy

Copyright © 2022 by S.L. Newman

All rights reserved. No part of this publication may be reproduced, stored or transmitted in any form or by any means, electronic, mechanical, photocopying, recording, scanning, or otherwise without written permission from the publisher. It is illegal to copy this book, post it to a website, or distribute it by any other means without permission.

S.L. Newman asserts the moral right to be identified as the author of this work.

S.L. Newman has no responsibility for the persistence or accuracy of URLs for external or third-party Internet Websites referred to in this publication and does not guarantee that any content on such Websites is, or will remain, accurate or appropriate.

Designations used by companies to distinguish their products are often claimed as trademarks. All brand names and product names used in this book and on its cover are trade names, service marks, trademarks and registered trademarks of their respective owners. The publishers and the book are not associated with any product or vendor mentioned in this book. None of the companies referenced within the book have endorsed the book.

First edition

This book was professionally typeset on Reedsy.
Find out more at reedsy.com

Contents

1

Introduction

Have you ever said or heard someone say, "I wish I had his/her energy"? Usually, this statement is made when watching children at play. Their energy appears endless. Can you recall the energy you had as a child? Can you remember waking up on Saturday mornings bright eyed and bushy tailed and bouncing out of bed? You could not wait to start the day! The possibilities for the day were endless and you had all the energy necessary to engage in any opportunities that came your way. In fact, you had so much energy, your parents had to tell you to go to bed.

Oh, how times have changed! As we get older, it seems our energy drains more and more with each passing year. We no longer bounce out of bed but instead hit the snooze button to avoid getting out of bed. Instead of being told to go to bed, we look forward to bedtime and usually collapse in bed completely exhausted.

What happened? Surely, we are not meant to go through our days feeling exhausted and worn down. Twenty-year-olds now have complaints of fatigue and burnout. Twenty-year-olds!

If you are sick and tired of feeling so darn tired, then this is the book for you. You can feel energetic again, ready to conquer the day. You do not have to wake-up every morning feeling like you don't have the energy to get everything done then collapse into bed each night from sheer exhaustion. With a few simple tweaks, you can increase your energy each and every day no matter what is on your agenda.

The strategies in this book are simple but that does not necessarily mean they are easy. One of the primary reasons we feel so drained on a continuous basis is because of the habits we have that are zapping our energy instead of boosting our energy. Habits are not always easy to break or change. That is why a strategy may seem simple and common sense when you read it but is difficult to implement. Be patient with yourself! Change is never easy but it almost always worth it. Don't try to implement every strategy in this book at once. Make one or two changes at a time and build from there. After a few weeks, an amazing thing will happen. With each new habit that you implement, you will notice small increases in your energy level. This will motivate you to implement more new habits and kick the habits that are no longer serving you.

I would like you to begin with a simple exercise. Find a comfortable place you can sit quietly for 5-10 minutes. Close your eyes. Take 3 slow, deep breaths. Now visualize yourself with endless energy. See yourself waking up in the morning, ready to start your day and not hitting the snooze button. See yourself driving to work or driving the kids to school singing your favorite song with a smile on your face. Visualize yourself attacking your to do list for the day, whether it is work outside of the home or chores and errands you must complete. See yourself gliding through the day getting everything done that needs to be completed and doing so with grace and ease. Try to see your face and body going through the motions and feel the energy flowing through you. See yourself coming home at the end of the day and walking through the door ready to greet your spouse, kids, family or pets. You are full of joy and peace and so grateful to spend time with those you love. You have energy to play with the kids or the dog. Maybe you decide to go for a walk or a run before dinner. See yourself doing the things you currently wish you had the energy to do. Finally, visualize yourself crawling into bed at the end of a completely ordinary but wonderful day. You feel calm, relaxed and sleepy but not exhausted. You are satisfied with the day. You lay your head on the pillow and look forward to a great night's sleep. Truly see yourself going through your day with boundless energy and feel what that would be like for you.

With the right tools this can be your reality. Let's get started!

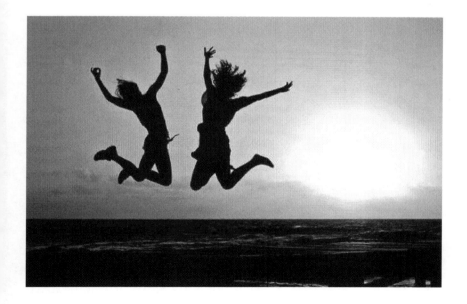

2

Food as fuel

Too often we look at food and think "what do I want to eat" instead of asking "what does my body need"? I want you to think of your body as a gorgeous high-end sports car. You know the one- your dream car. The car that most of us can't afford but certainly can dream about. Now you would never even consider filling the fuel tank with regular unleaded or performing a DIY oil change on that car would you? Of course not! You know what goes into the car determines its performance and longevity. The same is true for you. You are a gorgeous high-end human being, and you deserve to treat yourself accordingly. What you put into your body each and every day determines your performance so why not fuel your body the best way you possible can?

This is not a diet plan. I am not going to tell you what to eat or how often to eat in order to lose weight and gain energy. I am going to tell you how the foods you choose to eat effect your energy levels. It's up to you to decide which changes you want to make.

Sometimes when we are tired, we reach to food to give us energy.

This is not a bad habit to have but the foods you choose can have the reverse effect and drain your energy instead of giving you an energy boost. Below are some common foods and food groups that may be zapping your energy without you knowing it.

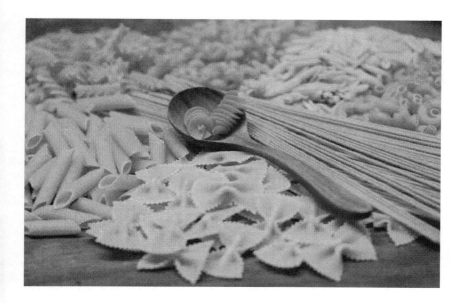

1. White bread, pasta and rice- all whole grain kernels contain 3 parts- the bran, the germ and the endosperm. Each part contains important nutrients that can affect your energy levels. The bran is the fiber rich outer layer that contains B vitamins and nutrients. The germ is the nutrient packed core that is rich in healthy fats, vitamin E, B vitamins and antioxidants. The endosperm is the interior layer that contains carbohydrates, proteins and a small number of vitamins and minerals. B vitamins have a direct impact on your energy levels, brain function and cell metabolism.

Unfortunately, during the refining process of grain, most of the bran and some of the germ are removed. This results in loss of dietary fiber, vitamins and minerals. In addition, refined grains have a higher starch content than whole grains. Processed grains are digested much faster than whole grains and are absorbed more quickly. A meal high in processed grains may cause a spike in blood sugar and insulin levels. You may experience a short burst in energy following one of these meals but that is usually followed by an energy drain and feeling like you need a nap.

2. Yogurts, breakfast cereals and other morning favorites with added sugar- like processed grains, foods high in sugar can cause a spike in blood sugar and insulin levels. It is common to crave high sugar breakfast cereals first thing in the morning because you are looking for that energy boost. Some popular breakfast cereals derive as much as 50% of the total carbs straight from added sugar. No doubt that will give you the energy boost you are looking for. What you weren't expecting was the energy drain you will feel a few hours later. In addition, studies have shown that starting the day off with a high sugar meal can cause you to crave more high sugar foods throughout the day. So, if you start the day with a high sugar cereal for breakfast, you might be hungry 2 hours later and decide to have a healthy snack like yogurt. Unfortunately, the yogurt you chose also has added sugar. If this continues throughout the day you will find yourself in an energy depleting cycle that initially provides the boost you are craving but quickly leaves you feeling drained. Breakfast may be one the most difficult times to detect foods with added sugar because we all grew up eating cereal, yogurt, juice, muffins, and granola bars as part of a normal breakfast.

3. Alcohol- there can be a lot of emotion associated with this category. Some people end the day with a drink to relieve stress and relax. Once that stress is relieved a person may feel their energy has

been restored. This may be true for you, but it can also be an energy zapper for others. Alcohol could reduce your motivation to get things done. It literally can suck the energy right out of you. Of course, alcohol effects everyone differently. One drink may provide an energy drain for one person and a motivational boost for another. Studies have shown that consuming high quantities of alcohol close to bedtime does effect sleep quality. A decrease in sleep quality can cause you to begin the day feeling drained and not well rested. Low to moderate levels of alcohol consumption are considered one or fewer drinks per day for women and two or fewer drinks a day for men, according to the CDC. A drink is defined as 12 ounces of beer, 5 ounces of wine or 1.5 ounces of spirits.

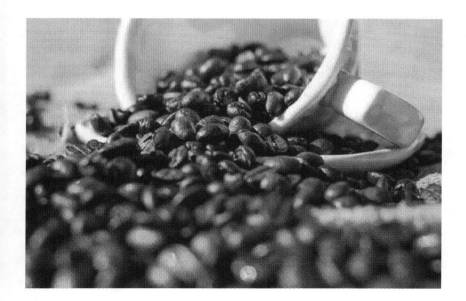

1. Coffee- I know what you are thinking, coffee gives me energy!! While this may be true for most people most of the time, too much of a good thing can have the opposite effect. In moderation, coffee can provide a quick burst of energy and even improve brain function. Coffee contains caffeine and too much caffeine or caffeine consumed at the wrong time can be an energy drain. The biggest concern around coffee is how much are you consuming and how close to bedtime are you having a cup of joe. Too much caffeine has a direct impact on your quality of sleep. Poor sleep quality leads to waking up tired and feeling like you tossed and turned all night. Repeating a high coffee consumption daily puts you into a vicious cycle of poor sleep, waking up feeling exhausted so you consume more coffee, and so on. Caffeine works like a drug-over time your body requires more caffeine to get the same burst of energy. Coffee does have positive physical and mental effects, so you don't have to cut it out completely. If you are drinking more than 4 cups of coffee per day currently, start with limiting yourself to just 4 cups per day. After a few weeks, drop that to 3 cups per day, then 2 cups per day with the last cup of coffee being consumed no closer than 6-8 hours before bedtime.

2. Energy drinks- energy drinks are a double whammy. Most energy drinks are high in sugar and caffeine. We have already discussed the negative effects of both, but let's quickly review. While sugar can provide a quick energy boost, it also spikes blood sugar and insulin levels. Following this spike, you could feel tired and drained. Some energy drinks contain as much as 10 teaspoons of sugar! In addition to the high sugar content, energy drinks may have high caffeine levels. A standard cup of coffee (8 oz) contains approximately 100mg of caffeine. There are energy drinks on the market that contain up to 400mg of caffeine- that is 4 times the amount in coffee. You may be thinking this increased caffeine level

will give you just the energy boost you are looking for. However, such high levels of caffeine may have negative side effects such as heart palpitations, anxiety and jitteriness. Not all energy drinks are bad, but the key is to know what you are consuming. Read the labels and look at the sugar and caffeine content.

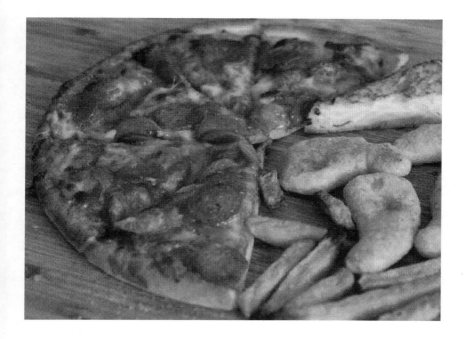

1. Fried and fast foods- when we are tired, the last thing we want to think about is what to eat so we tend to go for a quick and easy meal. In America, you can find a fast-food restaurant on almost any street corner. In most cases, those fast foods are fried foods. Unfortunately, choosing fried foods can leave you feeling more tired. Fried and fast foods are not nutrient dense foods and are

usually high in fat. The high fat content effects digestion as well. When food takes longer to digest, the increase in energy from a meal is delayed. Consuming too many fatty foods at a meal can also lead to feeling overly full. As a result, you may feel less motivated to get anything done.

2. Low calorie foods- while low calorie foods do have a place in our diets, too many low-calorie foods throughout the day can completely zap your energy. A calorie is literally a unit of energy. The calories from food provide your body with the energy it needs to perform the basic functions to keep you alive- breathing, heart beating, thinking. Depending on your age, gender, height, weight and activity level, your basal metabolic rate could be anywhere from 1200 calories/day to 2800 calories/day. A diet high in low calorie foods will not provide you with the energy you need to perform daily tasks. A significant decrease in calories can slow your metabolism and cause a hormonal imbalance which both cause fatigue.

You may be saying to yourself, "So what do I eat?" Advertising and marketing have conditioned consumers to believe that the foods listed previously are the go-to foods and beverages that will give us the energy needed to start the day or pull us through the post lunch blahs. What is interesting is that most of the foods that truly give us energy without negative side effects have amazing nutritional value overall. Using the analogy of a high-performance race car, think of the foods below as high octane fuel.

1. Brown rice- brown rice contains manganese. Manganese is a mineral that aides the body in producing energy from carbohy-

drates. The higher the manganese the longer your energy levels stay elevated following a meal. In addition, brown rice is a complex carbohydrate, so it takes the body longer to digest than a simple carbohydrate. This results in a gradual increase in blood sugar at opposed to a rapid spike followed by an energy drain. Complex carbs provide a consistent supply of energy throughout the day.

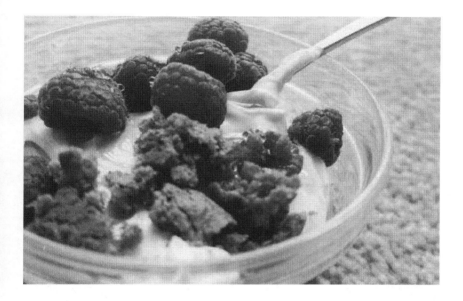

1. Greek yogurt- yogurt was mentioned previously as a food to avoid due to high sugar content, Greek yogurt is an exception. Greek yogurt does not contain high levels of added sugar. Greek yogurt is high in protein which slows digestion, keeps you full longer and provides a steady supply of energy. You can add fruit, nuts or unsweetened coconut flakes if the thought of eating plain yogurt is unappealing.

2. Beans- beans are an amazing source of energy. They are high in fiber, protein and B vitamins. The high fiber content of beans slows digestion in the stomach which makes you feel fuller longer. As mentioned earlier, protein takes longer to digest than carbohydrates which helps in providing a steady state of energy. Since beans are high in both fiber and protein, they are excellent sources of consistent steady levels of energy. Pair beans with brown rice and you will have a power packed meal.

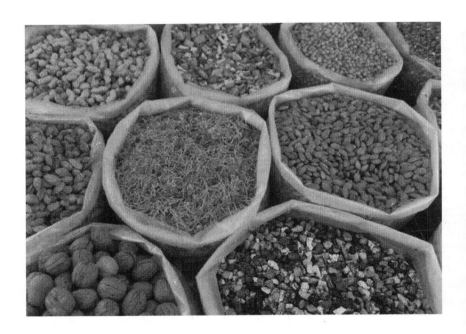

1. Nuts- nuts are a great on-the-go snack to keep energy up between meals. Nuts are high in unsaturated fat and protein so you will feel satisfied and energized. Try walnuts, almonds, cashews, pistachios, or hazelnuts. You may even want to add some dried fruit and

create your own trail mix. It is important to keep an eye on the serving size though since nuts can be high in calories.

2. Oranges- most people know oranges are high in Vitamin C. What some people don't know is vitamin C helps reduce oxidative stress in the body and reduce fatigue. Oranges are also high in potassium. Low levels of potassium in the body can result in fatigue. Oranges help increase potassium levels. Oranges also contain folate or folic acid which is one of the B vitamins. All B vitamins help convert food into fuel. For an additional boost, try adding vanilla protein powder to fresh squeezed orange juice for a delicious smoothie.

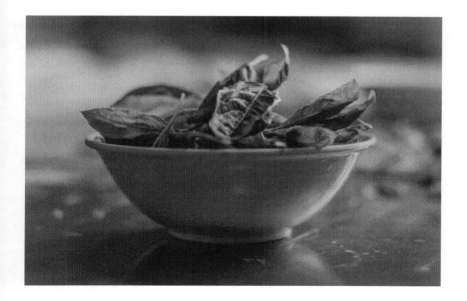

1. Spinach- spinach is considered by many to be a superfood. It is an amazing source of iron, nutrients and tyrosine. Low levels of iron can leave you feeling fatigues throughout the day. Per 100g, spinach contains the same amount of iron as meat. Spinach is high in fiber, vitamin C, folate and potassium. The benefits of these nutrients were discussed previously. Tyrosine is an amino acid which helps improve alertness, attention and focus. Can you see why spinach has been called a superfood? Not everyone can stomach a spinach salad or serving of steamed spinach though. An alternative could be placing a handful of spinach in a smoothie with fresh or frozen fruit. It is delicious and you won't even taste the spinach.

2. Quinoa- though technically a seed, quinoa is classified as a whole grain. It is high in protein and fiber. As mentioned earlier, this combination keeps you feeling full longer and provides a steady release of energy throughout the day. Quinoa is also high in amino acids, magnesium, folate and manganese which all play a role in energy production in the body. Try quinoa as a side dish or added to your favorite salad.

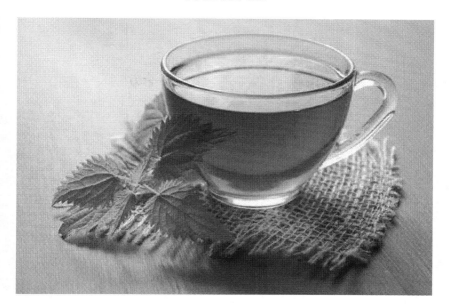

1. Green tea- green tea is an excellent alternative to coffee or energy drinks. Green tea still contains caffeine, but the levels are nowhere near those found in some energy drinks. You will get the benefits of caffeine without the side effects of excessive levels. Green tea can be consumed hot or iced. If you need to add some sweetener, try a small amount of honey or stevia.

3

Exercise and Movement

I know what you are thinking- if you are tired, exhausted and completely drained of energy, how the heck are you going to be motivated to exercise? I see the irony but trust me, exercise does make you more energetic. The biggest hurdle you will face is taking that first step to get moving. It's kind of like a car building speed from a complete stop. It takes a few seconds to get up to speed but once the car gets moving, it just coasts right along. Whether you choose to exercise first thing in the morning, on your lunch break or in the evening, try to find a way to motivate yourself to get going. This may mean laying your exercise clothes out the night before, so you are ready to go first thing in the morning or heading straight to the gym after work before you get bogged down with the responsibilities of home.

Exercise releases endorphins and endorphins are the body's "feel good" hormones. You may have heard of the "runner's high" that some runners experience. Well, this is due to high endorphin levels caused by exercise, in this case running. Fortunately, for those of us who aren't so crazy about running, we can experience this same endorphin release from any form of exercise that requires a burst of energy.

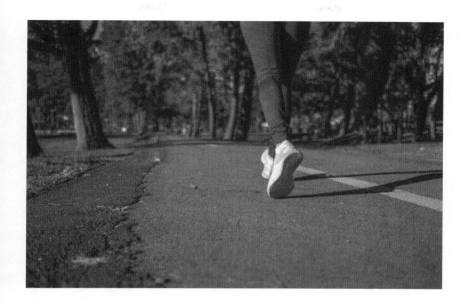

1. One of the simplest and most convenient forms of exercise is walking. It literally can be done anywhere with no equipment necessary, and we all have the skills required! Walking increases the heart rate and respiratory rate but is a low- impact activity that is easy on the joints. A 30-minute walk can help improve your overall physical fitness, help clear your mind and improve well-being and improve your mood. If you can't commit to 30 minutes a day, start with 10 minutes. Maybe a 10-minute walk at lunch or a walk around the block with the family after dinner. Doing something is better than doing nothing so start where you can. Once you realize the benefits of walking and experience how good you feel, you may want to increase the time to 30 minutes or

even longer.

2. Swimming is another wonderful low-impact exercise. Swimming laps is a great cardiovascular exercise, but it is not the only option. Water aerobics can be done in almost any size pool and can be done with or without equipment. Swimming laps and water aerobics can be done at your own pace and are gentle on your joints and back. Try taking the plunge first thing in the morning if possible. The cool, refreshing water will give you a burst of energy.

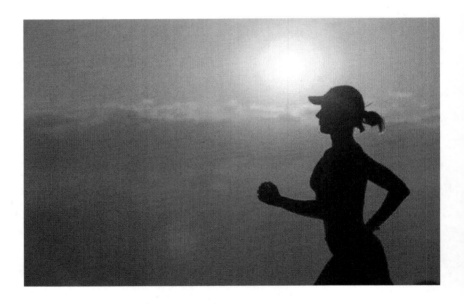

1. As mentioned earlier, running is a great exercise option. Running or jogging is not for everyone since it can be very hard on the joints and lower back. However, for those that feel walking is not strenuous enough for them, jogging may be the solution. Since jogging is an aerobic activity, your heart, lungs and muscles will all

benefit. Another benefit to jogging is the mental clarity following a run. Some runners report getting into the zone during a run where they are aware of their surroundings but their mind is completely clear, almost blank. At the end of the run, they feel refreshed and have mental clarity similar to meditation.

2. Do you remember as a child, riding your bicycle for hours and hours? You could ride all day and never get tired. Why not try it again? Cycling is another low-impact exercise that can be done almost anywhere. It does require equipment of course but there are bikes for every budget. If you live close to work, maybe you could bike to and from work every day. Or maybe you gather the family and head out for a ride in the evening or on weekends. Have fun! Don't forget about indoor cycling or spin classes. There are so many different bikes and programs to choose from nowadays that you can find the perfect fit for you. You may want to take spin classes at the local gym or invest in your own bike and sign up for classes through Peloton, Bowflex or NordicTrack.

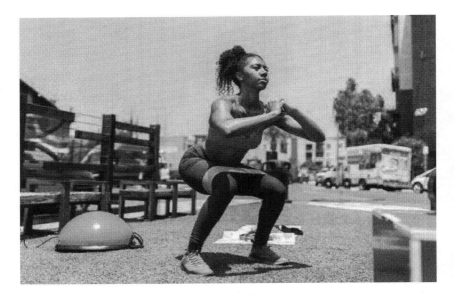

1. Weight training can benefit anyone at any age. You do not have to lift heavy weights to obtain the benefits of weight training either. Body weight activities such as squats, push-ups, pull-ups, lunges and dips can be just as beneficial. Not everyone has access to a gym or has a home gym in the garage or basement and that's okay. It does not take much to get started. Try doing 10 push-ups or 20 squats first thing in the morning. Knock out 20 lunges after lunch. Maybe get the family involved since no equipment is required and set up a circuit everyone can do- 10 push-ups, 5 pull-ups, 20 squats, 20 crunches, 20 lunges, 10 dips for example.

2. Yoga is an excellent exercise option for anyone. The mental and physical benefits of yoga will leave you feeling calm and rejuvenated. Yoga is a practice, and everyone is on their own journey so there is no reason to feel intimidated or apprehensive. There are several different types of yoga from hatha to power to aerial and everything in between. Explore the different options

and find one that works for you. Yoga should give you a sense of wellbeing and restoration so search for the yoga practice that is best for your personality and fitness level. You could find a yoga class locally or search online for thousands of free classes.

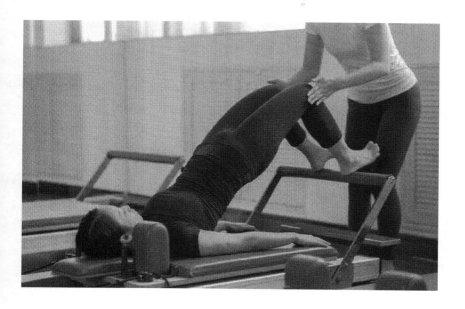

1. Pilates was first created in in the 1920's by Joseph Pilates for the purpose of rehabilitation. In was created to strengthen the body and heal aches and pains. Dealing with aches and pains on a continuous basis can be a constant drain on our energy. We get sick and tired of feeling sick and tired and seldom have the energy to deal with daily activities. If this is the case for you, Pilates may be the answer to getting you started on an exercise program. Pilates is low-impact, easy on the joints and back, can be done in a small space in the convenience of your own home and can be done

with or without equipment. Pilates is a total body workout that increases core strength, improves posture, decreases back pain, increases energy, decreases stress and reduces menstrual pain.

No matter which activity you choose, the important thing is to get moving. Start small if you have to with 10-15 minutes a day and build up from there. Any movement is better than no movement at all. On the difficult days when you truly do not feel like working out, give yourself 5 minutes before you decide today is not the day. Five minutes of movement, whatever it is, and if you still do not want to exercise, then stop and try again tomorrow. Over time, if you stick with it, exercise will be something you look forward to because you know how good you are going to feel, physically, mentally and emotionally when you are done. Be honest with yourself but also be patient. We all know exercise is good for us for numerous reasons. This is not earth shattering news. Our goal is to boost our energy and keep it elevated so we can live the life we want to live. Allow that to be your motivation every day. Remind yourself that you want to have the energy to play with your kids or grandkids, you want to have the energy to be present for your spouse or significant other at the end of the day, you want to have the energy to go back to school to get a better education so you can land a higher paying job. Whatever your reason is for wanting more energy to get through the day, let that be your motivation to get moving (literally) for 20-30 minutes daily.

Before starting any exercise program, be sure to consult with your physician to review and medical conditions or concerns that you may have.

4

Decision fatigue

D ecision fatigue is defined as the inability or decreased capacity of an individual to make decisions due to brain fatigue caused by having to make too many decisions throughout the day. While there is little to no scientific evidence that decision fatigue is a real thing, most people can relate to the statement "If I have to make one more decision today, I swear I am going to scream!". We begin making decisions as soon as we wake up in the morning such as what to eat for breakfast and what to wear to work. According to Psychology Today, a person can make as many as 35,000 decisions over the course of the day! Thirty-five thousand decisions! No wonder we are all so tired. Mental exhaustion can progress to physical exhaustion and lack of energy. As the day goes on, a person is required to make more and more decisions which can cause a person to feel drained mentally and physically.

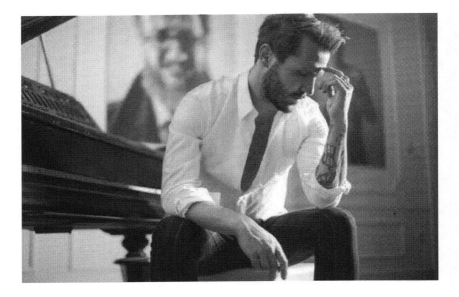

Fortunately, there are some things you can do to combat and even prevent decision fatigue.

1. Make important decisions first. If each decision we make reduces our energy for future decisions, then it would make sense to make the big or important decisions when our energy is at its highest level.

2. Remove distractions. When you decide to work on a project or complete a task, remove all distractions that will pull you in another direction. Set your cell phone on do not disturb or turn the ringer off. Close all windows on your computer except those needed to complete the task you are working on. Turn the TV off so you aren't tempted to glance in its direction.

3. Plan meals. Whether you meal plan and prep for the week or simply plan dinners ahead of time, removing this decision making process can be a game changer. By planning meals in advance, you eliminate having to decide under pressure. It can be stressful to

decide where to go for lunch when you have a limited amount of time or trying to decide what's for dinner after a long and grueling day at work. A bonus to meal planning is that you tend to make healthier choices of the foods you eat which has a direct impact on your energy level.

4. Take breaks. If you are mentally exhausted and simply cannot make one more decision, take a break. It can be 5-10 minutes. A 5–10-minute break allows your mind to reset and refresh. You may want to sit quietly for 5-10 minutes. Mindlessly scroll through social media. Watch a quick video on YouTube. Take a walk outside. Do whatever works for you. The point is to pull you away temporarily from the activity that is mentally draining you.

5. Plan tomorrow today. An excellent way to decrease the number of decisions you must make in a day is to plan your day the night before. Time block your day into half hour or one hour increments, you can use a day planner for this or simple piece of paper. Then write down all the activities you need to complete the following day. If there are items you need to gather for an activity such as gym clothes, the kid's baseball equipment, or snacks for an office party, gather those items up before you go to bed and place them by the door. Now your brain is not wasting energy first thing in the morning trying to remember what you need to bring. Review the activities for the day and make sure none of them overlap or are scheduled so closely that you will not be able to arrive on time. Rushing from place to place or realizing you scheduled yourself to be in two places at the same time causes unnecessary stress which is an enormous drain on your energy. You can take this a step further and time block your day for certain activities. Divide the day up into 2-, 3- or 4-hour blocks then assign a specific activity to each block. Pencil in meals accordingly and assign at least 30 minutes for some sort of physical activity. For instance, one block

could be top priority work or the important and urgent tasks of the day. Another block could be for meetings or group collaboration. Another block could be for organizing or accounting task that need to be completed daily. If each hour(s) of your day has an assigned purpose, you no longer must decide what you should be doing next. The decision is already made for you. In addition, your mind does not wander off and begin thinking about other activities because it knows there is an assigned time for that task. You can completely focus on the task at hand.

5

Ahhhhhh Sleep!

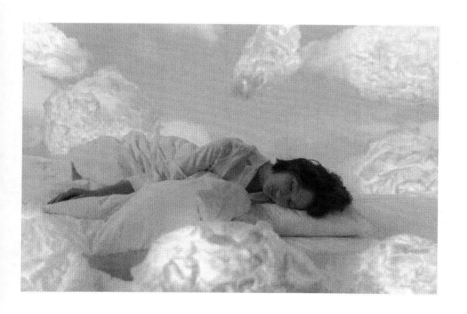

When was the last time you had a real good night's sleep? The kind of sleep where you felt like as soon as your head hit the pillow, you closed your eyes and fell into a deep sleep. When you woke the next morning, you weren't sure if you moved a single muscle all night and you felt full of energy and ready to take on the day! If you are like most people, it's been months or even years since you have experienced that kind of rest.

There are many reasons that most of us are tossing and turning instead of falling asleep quickly and staying asleep through the night. Some of the more common explanations are: too much caffeine or alcohol too close to bedtime, shift work, jet lag, stress, eating too close to bedtime or eating the wrong foods before bed, sleep disorders like sleep apnea or restless leg syndrome, or drug side effects that disrupt sleep.

Getting a goodnight's sleep in just as important as eating the right foods and getting exercise when it comes to increasing your energy. Not getting enough sleep or poor sleep quality effects your hormones, brain function and physical performance in addition to zapping your energy. Fortunately, there are some tips and tricks you can implement to ensure you are getting the best rest possible.

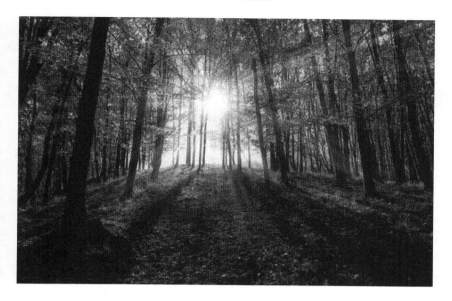

1. Let the sunshine in! Have you heard of circadian rhythm? It is the body's natural time clock and one of its functions is to tell you when to stay awake and when to go to sleep. Circadian rhythms are naturally tied to the cycle of day and night. Light exposure causes the body to send signals to the brain to generate alertness which keeps you awake and active. As the sun goes down and night appears, the body releases melatonin, a hormone that encourages sleep and we begin to feel tired and our mind slows down. Inadequate exposure to bright light can disrupt the circadian rhythm and effect sleep quality. The good news is, you don't have to spend hours outside to see the benefits of light exposure and align your circadian rhythm. Studies have shown that just 2 hours of bright light exposure during the day can improve sleep quality and duration. If daily exposure to sunlight is not an option try artificial bright light devices or bulbs, they can be just as effective.

2. Watch out for the blue light. Blue light is emitted in large amounts from smartphones, tablets and computers. Using these devices right before bed disrupts your circadian rhythm because your body confuses the blue light with bright light. Melatonin production is affected since your body still thinks it's daytime and that directly impacts your sleep quality. While not watching TV and turning off all devices at least 2 hours before bedtime is ideal, it is not always practical. There are a few things to try to decrease blue light exposure before bed. Try wearing glasses that block blue light when using your phone, tablet or computer. These can be found easily online and are relatively inexpensive. Download an app on your tablet or computer to block blue light such as Iris Mini, Redshift, SunsetScreen or Night Shift. You can do the same thing on your smartphone. Simply go into the app store and search for blue light blocker or blue light filter and several options will come up.

3. Curb the caffeine. As we discussed in the section on using food as fuel, coffee, consumed too close to bedtime can have devastating effects on sleep quality. Energy drinks and other caffeinated beverages can have the same effect. Caffeine levels in the body can stay elevated for up to 8 hours following consumption. Those elevated levels stimulate your nervous system and brain activity which can prevent you from falling asleep or cause you to wake after only a few hours of rest. Some experts say not to consume caffeine after 2:00/3:00 in the afternoon. Since not everyone goes to bed at the same time, this advice does not apply to every person. However, you should limit caffeine consumption to 6-8 hours before bedtime for caffeine levels to decrease and not interfere with sleep.

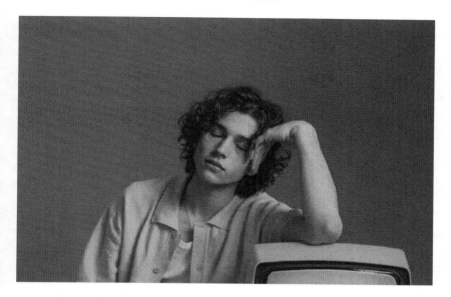

1. Know when to nap. Do you remember taking a nap as a kid? Sure you may have fought laying down and taking a nap (you didn't want to miss anything) but when you woke up, you were full of energy and ready to get back to playing. Naps have a place and a purpose and can be extremely rejuvenating. A power nap is commonly defined as a short sleep (20-30 minutes) that terminates before deep sleep and leaves a person feeling energized. The issue occurs when napping is irregular, or naps extend beyond 30 minutes and a person falls into a deep sleep. Irregular napping and long naps can decrease sleep quality at night because both effect the internal clock. This in turn effects circadian rhythm. As mentioned above, an aligned circadian rhythm promotes a good night's sleep. If you enjoy afternoon naps, try setting an alarm so you don't exceed 20-30 minutes.

2. Rise and shine!! Just like the cycle of day and night, light and dark, effect your circadian rhythm, so does the time you go to

sleep and wake each day. Your body loves predictability and consistency. Going to bed at the same time each night and waking at the same time each morning, creates a pattern that is consistent and predictable. This is when your body gets in the zone. Ideally, you should allow your body to wake on its own each day. For most of us, this would mean rolling out of bed around 9 or 10 o'clock. Not exactly the best plan if we are expected at work by 8am. Start with setting an alarm to go off at the same time every day, yes weekends too. If the same time on weekdays and weekends is too aggressive, try waking at the same time on weekdays then push back you're alarm no more than 3 hours on weekends. The goal is to create consistency and predictability. Don't worry about what time you go to bed. Eventually, your body will adjust to the new wake up time and naturally fall into a pattern for bedtime.

3. Elevate your environment. There are a few key factors to consider when setting up the perfect environment for a good night's sleep. External lights, noise, temperature and furniture placement all have a direct effect on the quality and duration of sleep. Many experts agree that a temperature between 60-71 degrees Fahrenheit, with 65 degrees being ideal, is advisable for most people. This may seem a bit extreme for some but consider this, your body temperature drops naturally while you sleep which makes you feel drowsy. Lowering the temperature in the room helps sustain a low core temperature. Play around with the temperature to find what works best. Remember, you can add a blanket or comforter, remove a layer of bedding or wear warmer or cooler bedclothes.

Loud or unusual noises can greatly disrupt sleep by keeping you awake entirely or causing you to wake up intermittently throughout the night. Depending on where you live, you may have no control over the noises you hear at night. Luckily, there are some options to decrease external noise so you can get some rest. One option is noise blocking curtains or inserts which can result in a 50-70% noise reduction. Another option is a white noise machine or listening to soothing music as you fall asleep. Anything that can help mask other sounds and allow you to relax. A relatively inexpensive option is a simple floor fan. The whirring sound of the fan can drown out other noises and has a similar effect to a white noise machine.

We have already discussed the effect of light and sleep and the impact light has on circadian rhythm. Be mindful of the light sources in the bedroom and the intensity prior to bedtime. Remember to block blue light if you are using devices prior to going to sleep. If you like to read in bed, use a warm or amber light instead of a natural or bright light.

In makes sense that cozy sheets, a soft pillow and fluffy comforter can aide in getting a good night's sleep, but have you ever considered how your furniture in the bedroom is arranged? According to Sleep Junkie, a website devoted to sleep science, it can make a big difference. They completed a survey of 1,000 participants regarding furniture arrangement in the bedroom and quality of sleep. To optimize sleep quality and duration, the best furniture placement, according to the survey is: a bed centered or an interior wall with the door on an adjacent wall, the TV across from the bed and a window to the side of the bed. This makes sense if you consider the effects of light and sleep that we discussed earlier. By placing the bed away from windows and doors, any light from outside or a hallway is diminished. A window to the side of the bed allows just enough natural light to filter in at the start of the day to allow you to wake naturally.

1. Create a routine. Following the same routine every night before you go to bed helps your body and mind prepare for bedtime. Don't overcomplicate this. Most people do the same or similar things

every night before going to bed but may not realize it. Setting up a bedtime routine makes steps more purposeful. The goal is to help you relax, unwind and let go of the day. Take a hot bath or shower. Have a light snack or herbal tea. Listen to music. Meditate. Do some light stretching. Read a book. Journal. It doesn't matter so much what you do as long as you do the same thing every night. Over time your mind learns that these are the activities you do to prepare for bed so you can relax and rest.

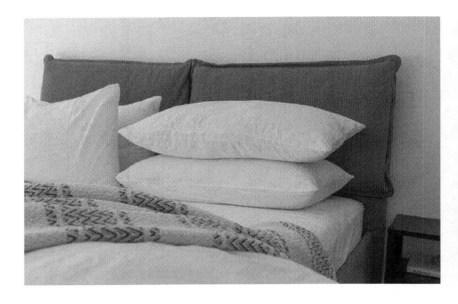

1. Comfort is key. How old is your mattress? When was the last time you replaced your pillow? It is recommended that you replace your pillow every 1-2 years and your mattress every 8-10 years. Try this: fold your pillow in half. Does it stay that way? Then it's time to get a new pillow. Not only do pillows wear down over

time but dead skin cells, hair and body oils build-up on the pillows surface. Replacing a pillow is a somewhat inexpensive investment. Replacing a mattress in a completely different story but can be well worth the investment. A poor quality or worn-out mattress can cause back pain, shoulder pain and back or neck stiffness. As a result, sleep quality decreases. If you just can't get comfortable at night and your bedding is beyond its life expectancy, consider replacing it.

2. Rule out a disorder. Not all sleep issues can be cured with the tips previously mentioned. Some people suffer from sleep disorders and don't know it. Sleep apnea, restless leg syndrome, insomnia, narcolepsy, non-24-hour sleep wake disorder are all common medical conditions that impair your ability to get a good night's sleep. If you or a family member believes you suffer from any of these conditions, please seek the advice of a medical professional. There is no need to continue to suffer. A sleep study can be performed to diagnose these conditions. Once diagnosed, your physician can begin to help you determine the best course of action so you can get the rest you deserve.

6

Supplements

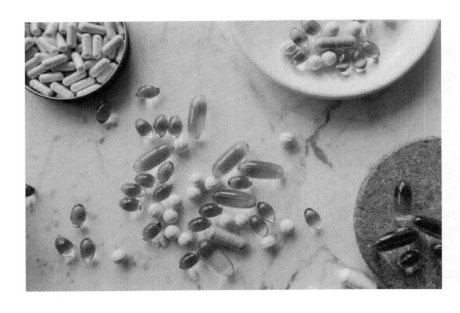

Y ou're eating the right foods, moving you body every day, getting enough rest but you still feel like you need an energy boost. Supplements may be the answer you're looking for. Here are a few vitamins and supplements that can help:

<u>Ashwagandha</u>- medicinal herb believed to reduce mental and physical fatigue and increase energy levels

<u>Rhodiola Rosea</u>- herb that is believed to enhance the body's ability to adapt to stress therefore reducing fatigue caused by stress

<u>B12</u>- vitamin that helps convert the food you eat into energy that is used by the cells. B12 deficiency causes fatigue and weakness. Older adults, persons with GI disorders and vegans/vegetarians may be at risk for B12 deficiency.

<u>Iron</u>- iron deficiency can result in anemia which causes fatigue and weakness. Iron comes from the food we eat and is used to make hemoglobin which carries oxygen throughout the body. Those who are pregnant, eat a diet low in iron or have heavy blood loss from a period or internal bleeding can be at risk.

<u>CoQ10</u>- coenzyme Q10 is made naturally in the body and is used by the cells to make energy and protect themselves from damage. Low levels of CoQ10 lead to decreased energy production by the cells which leads to fatigue. CoQ10 levels decrease with age and medical conditions such as cancer and diabetes or those who take statins.

These are just a few of the supplements that are available to help increase energy levels. Before taking any supplement, consult with your physician. He/she may want to complete bloodwork to determine any deficiencies. Supplements can interact with prescribed medication, so it is crucial that your physician know what you are taking.

7

Conclusion

I t is not possible to turn back time and be a child again. However, it is possible to have the same energy you had as a child and soar through the day with unlimited energy.

Please don't feel you must make every change or implement every suggestion in this book. That would be overwhelming. Instead, pick one or two changes you feel comfortable making and start with those. Maybe it's cutting down on the number of energy drinks you drink daily or replacing a fast-food hamburger at lunch with a grilled chicken sandwich. Think baby steps. Once you are comfortable with those changes, you introduce a few more. Each choice you make to eliminate foods that drain your energy, introduce foods that increase your energy, move your body and clear your mind will have a snowball effect on your energy level. The changes may be small at first, so small you may not really notice them. However, the longer you continue to implement the changes and build new habits, the more noticeable the changes will be. You'll realize you no longer craze that afternoon shot of caffeine or feel like you need a nap every afternoon to make it through the day.

You deserve to live an energetic and vivacious life doing the things you enjoy. My sincerest prayer for you is that by making a few small changes in how you fuel your body, relax your mind and move your body through exercise will give you the energy boost you are looking for. Cheers to unlimited energy!

If you found this book helpful, I'd be very appreciative if you left a favorable review for the book on Amazon!

8

Resources

Petre, A. (2018, February 18). *7 Foods the Drain.* Healthline. Retrieved July 31, 2022, from https://www.healthline.com/nutrition/foods-that-drain-energy#TOC_TITLE_HDR_8

Harvard T. H. Chan. (2019). *Whole Grains.* Harvard. Retrieved July 31, 2022, from https://www.hsph.harvard.edu/nutritionsource/what-should-you-eat/whole-grains/#:~:text=All%20whole%20grain%20kernels%20contain,magnesium%2C%20antioxidants%2C%20and%20phytochemicals.

Oghbaei, M. (2016, January 29). *Effect of primary processing of cereals and legumes on its nutritional quality.* Taylor & Francis Online. Retrieved July 31, 2022, from https://www.tandfonline.com/doi/full/10.1080/23311932.2015.1136015#:~:text=The%20nutritional%20composition%20of%20whole,phenolic%20compounds%2C%20and%20phytic%20acid.

Lang, A. (2021, November 2). *Can certain foods give you an energy boost?* Healthline. Retrieved July 31, 2022, from https://www.healthline.com/nutrition/energy-boosting-foods#basics

Meredith, D. (2022, January 5). *8 everyday foods that help boost your energy.* Taste of Home. Retrieved July 31, 2022, from https://www.tast eofhome.com/collection/foods-that-give-you-energy/

Rodriguez, D. (2019, May 1). *Why exercise boosts mood and energy.* Everyday Health. Retrieved July 31, 2022, from https://www.everyday health.com/fitness/workouts/boost-your-energy-level-with-exercise. aspx

Sleep Health Foundation. (2020, March 10). *Common Causes of Inadequate Sleep.* Retrieved July 31, 2022, from https://www.sleeph ealthfoundation.org.au/common-causes-of-inadequate-sleep.html

Pacheco, D. (2022, June 17). *The Bedroom Environment.* Sleep Foundation. Retrieved July 31, 2022, from https://www.sleepfoun dation.org/bedroom-environment

Bennett, J. (2019, November 4). *How to arrange your bedroom for the best night's sleep.* Better Home & Gardens. Retrieved July 31, 2022, from https://www.bhg.com/news/arrange-bedroom-sleep/

White, M. A. (2020, July 6). *What is decision fatigue?* Medical News Today. Retrieved July 31, 2022, from https://www.medicalnewstoday.c om/articles/decision-fatigue

Krockow, E. M. (2018, September 27). *How many decisions do we make each day?* Psychology Today. Retrieved July 31, 2022, from https://ww w.psychologytoday.com/us/blog/stretching-theory/201809/how-man y-decisions-do-we-make-each-day

Made in the USA
Columbia, SC
10 October 2022

69256823R00026